TRANSFORM YOUR LIFE WITH VAGUS NERVE MAGIC

Unleashing the Power Within to Reset, Activate, and Triumph Over Anxiety, Depression, Stress, Inflammation, while Amplifying Your Inherent Ability to Heal and Ignite a Journey of Wholeness and Wellness."

DR. MARIA MARTIN

Table of contents

Introduction

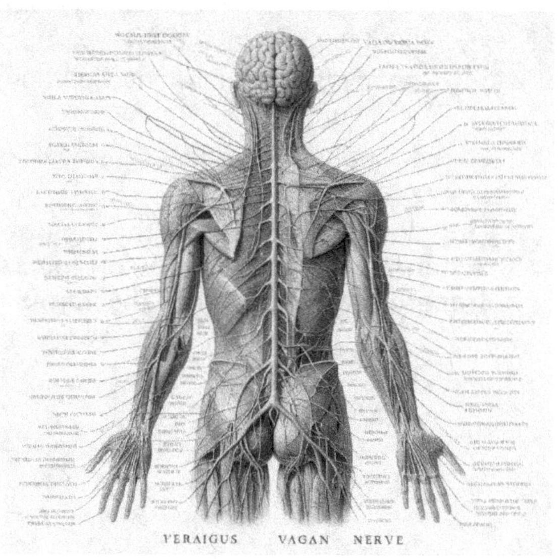

The vagus nerve is a hidden jewel within the complicated network of our neurological system. The vagus nerve, sometimes known as the "wandering nerve," plays an important role in orchestrating a symphony of biological activities that affect both mental and physical health. This article delves into the vagus nerve's structure, functioning, and transforming potential to reset, activate, and triumph over a variety of difficulties, including anxiety and depression, as well as stress and inflammation.

A brief overview of the vagus nerve.

The vagus nerve, often known as the tenth cranial nerve, is a miracle of nature. This wandering nerve, which originates in the brainstem and extends like a complicated network of fibres throughout the body, regulates a wide range of processes. The vagus nerve is a quiet conductor, directing our autonomic nervous system's symphony by managing heart rhythm, assisting digestion, and affecting breathing rate.

Its name, "vagus," comes from the Latin word for "wandering," which accurately describes the meandering journey it follows through the body. The vagus nerve is divided into two branches: cranial and spinal, and it links the brain to essential organs including the heart, lungs, and digestive system. This sophisticated network of communication enables the vagus nerve to send information between the brain and numerous organs, which is critical for maintaining homeostasis.

Understanding Its Role in Mental and Physical Well-Being

As we learn more about the vagus nerve, it becomes clear that this apparently little nerve holds the key to unlocking our full potential for health and wellness. The vagus nerve's effect is based on the connectivity of mental and physical health.

Understanding Mental Wellbeing

The vagus nerve is being more acknowledged for its significant influence on mental health. According to research, vagus nerve stimulation may significantly improve anxiety and depression management. The vagus nerve promotes calm and relaxation by modifying the parasympathetic nervous system, which helps to counteract the frequently overpowering nature of anxiety and depression disorders.

Moreover, the vagus nerve regulates the body's stress response. In a world full of ongoing challenges and demands, the capacity to successfully navigate and manage stress is critical for mental health. The vagus nerve, by its complicated link to the brain, helps to reduce stress by encouraging a healthy autonomic nervous system response.

Impact on Physical Well-Being

Beyond its influence on mental health, the vagus nerve is essential for physical well-being. One of its notable contributions is to the field of inflammation. Inflammation, a common denominator in many health disorders, is inextricably related to the vagus nerve. The nerve's activation has been linked to a decrease in inflammatory markers, underlining its potential as a comprehensive strategy to treating inflammatory disorders.

Furthermore, the vagus nerve plays an important role in the gut-brain axis, which is a dynamic interaction between the digestive system and brain. The health of the gut has a direct influence on general well-being, affecting not just digestion but also immunity and mood. Understanding and fostering the vagus nerve's involvement in this complex link is critical to reaching maximum health.

In sum, understanding the vagus nerve is like having the key to a treasure box of health. Unlocking the mysteries of this roaming nerve gives people the skills they need to negotiate the complexity of contemporary life, boosting mental resilience and physical vigour.

As we go through this book, we will learn about the architecture and functioning of the vagus nerve, how it affects mental and physical health, and how to use it to achieve transformational well-being. The vagus nerve encourages us to reset, activate, and triumph over life's adversities, providing a road to healing and a journey toward wholeness and wellbeing.

Chapter 1

Revealing the Vagus Nerve: Anatomy and Relationships

The vagus nerve, sometimes known as the "wandering nerve," is a fascinating part of the human nervous system that is remarkable for its unique structure and essential roles. By exploring the structure and activities of the vagus nerve, this section seeks to shed light on its many mysteries and clarify the close relationship it has with the brain.

Overview of Vagus Nerve Anatomy

The vagus nerve, also known as the tenth cranial nerve in technical terminology, is a broad neurological route that emerges from the brainstem. The word "wandering," which comes from Latin, accurately characterises its wide branches that weave throughout the body. The vagus nerve, which is made up of cranial and spinal components, is a master regulator that controls autonomic processes that are not under conscious control.

Branches of the Brain and Spine

The vagus nerve splits into four major streams in its cranial form: the recurrent laryngeal, superior laryngeal, pharyngeal, and auricular nerves. These branches, which go from the external ear to the complex web of cranial nerves involved in hearing, perform a variety of tasks.

The spinal branches, which arise from the upper spinal cord, are involved in the regulation of autonomic functions and total vagus nerve functioning.

Wide-ranging Pathways

The vagus nerve sets off on an intriguing trip via the neck, chest, and belly, connecting with vital organs including the heart, lungs, and digestive system. The brain and essential organs may communicate in both directions thanks to this complex network, which enables the vagus nerve to operate as a bridge and coordinate body processes.

The Vagus Nerve's Functions

The parasympathetic and sympathetic branches of the autonomic nervous system are both influenced by the vagus nerve, which functions as a complex actor in this system. Gaining knowledge of its many roles might help one appreciate how crucial it is to preserving homeostasis.

Regulation of the Parasympathetic Nervous System

As the master regulator of the parasympathetic nervous system, the vagus nerve sets the tone for the body's rest-and-digest condition.

- **Heart Rate Regulation:** The vagus nerve reduces the heart rate by producing acetylcholine, which helps to maintain a healthy cardiovascular system.

- **Management of the Digestive System**: In order to facilitate digestion and the absorption of nutrients, the vagus nerve promotes smooth muscle activity in the gastrointestinal system.

- **Respiratory Control:** The vagus nerve, which controls inspiration and expiration to ensure ideal oxygen exchange, is a major player in controlling breathing patterns.

- **Release of Anti-Inflammatory Signals**: Anti-inflammatory signals are released in response to vagus nerve stimulation, which controls inflammation and immunological responses.

Modulation of the Sympathetic Nervous System

The vagus nerve, while mostly linked to the parasympathetic nervous system, also contributes to the body's "fight or flight" instincts by regulating sympathetic responses.

- **Stress Response Dampening**: In times of stress, activation of the vagus nerve counteracts the effects of the sympathetic nervous system, enabling a precisely calibrated stress response.

- **Autonomic Function Balance**: The vagus nerve is a vital regulator that maintains the equilibrium between the sympathetic and parasympathetic branches of the autonomic nervous system, which is necessary for good health.

Relationship between the Brain and the Vagus Nerve

The vagus nerve and the brain are physically close, yet their complex relationship affects higher-order cognitive processes, emotional states, and mental activities.

The Brain's "Information Highway" is the Vagus Nerve

- **Bidirectional Communication:** The vagus nerve is an essential conduit for information transfer and regulation of the body's reactions between the brain and other organs.

- **Emotional Regulation:** The vagus nerve affects mood and stress tolerance by acting on the limbic system, which in turn affects emotional regulation.

- **Memory and Learning**: Studies indicate that the release of neurotransmitters like acetylcholine, which are involved in memory and learning processes, is influenced by the vagus nerve.

- **Neuroplasticity and Adaptation**: The vagus nerve's influence on neuroplasticity highlights how it shapes the body's reactions to outside stimuli and helps it adjust to a changing environment.

Stimulation of the Vagus Nerve and Brain Health

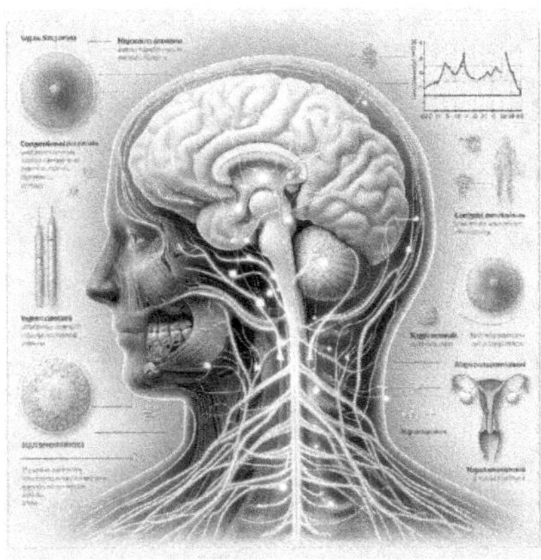

Potential for Therapeutic Interventions: Vagus nerve stimulation has shown promise in treating a range of neurological and psychiatric disorders by modifying brain activity.

- **Neuroprotective benefits:** Research indicates that stimulating the vagus nerve may have neuroprotective benefits, which might lessen the consequences of neurodegenerative illnesses.

Chapter 2

Revealing the Impact of the Vagus Nerve on Mental Wellbeing

More than just a conduit for physiological processes, the vagus nerve is a sophisticated neurological pathway that runs from the brainstem to several organs. It is essential in forming our mental and emotional health and is a major participant in the complex dance between the mind and body. We explore the substantial effects of the vagus nerve on mental health in this investigation, with particular attention to how it regulates anxiety and depression and how vagus nerve stimulation shows promise as a potent stress-reduction technique.

Part in the Handling of Anxiety and Depression

The vagus nerve is an unexpected interlocutor of anxiety and depression, two ubiquitous problems in today's fast-paced environment. With its vast network of connections, this wandering nerve is deeply woven into the emotional regulatory fabric and provides a unique means of treating various mental health issues.

- **Vagus Nerve and Emotional Control:**

The vagus nerve functions in the context of the autonomic nervous system, primarily affecting the parasympathetic branch. This system, often known as the "rest-and-digest" branch, is essential for controlling emotions. Managing anxiety and depression becomes especially dependent on the complex dance that the vagus nerve performs with the limbic system, the brain's emotional core.

▪ The Parasympathetic Nervous System Modification:

The vagus nerve's capacity to regulate the sympathetic nervous system, which is often hyperactive during the "fight-or-flight" reaction, is essential to understanding its function in mental health. The vagus nerve promotes calmness and relaxation by producing acetylcholine, which dampens excessive excitability in the brain.

▪ Neurotransmitter equilibrium:

Neurotransmitter imbalances, including those involving dopamine and serotonin, are often linked to anxiety and depression. The vagus nerve helps to maintain a delicate balance by influencing the release of neurotransmitters. Elevated serotonin production has been associated with vagus nerve stimulation, which has a favourable effect on mood and mental health.

- **Study Findings:**

The relationship between vagus nerve activity and mental health outcomes has been studied scientifically. Research indicates that those with greater vagal tone—a sign of robust vagus nerve function—are more resilient to stress and have a lower chance of developing anxiety and depression.

- **Uses in Clinical Practice:**

Novel treatment techniques have been prompted by the discovery of the vagus nerve's function in emotional regulation. Treatment options for severe depression and refractory anxiety disorders include vagus nerve stimulation (VNS), which involves using a device to administer electrical impulses to the vagus nerve. This modality emphasises the vagus nerve's practical effects on mental health, which go beyond theoretical ideas.

How Stress Is Reduced by Vagus Nerve Stimulation

Stress has become a ubiquitous companion in today's hectic world, impacting both mental and physical health. In the fight against stress, the vagus nerve—often hailed as the body's natural stress regulator—becomes an effective ally. Gaining knowledge about the mechanics of vagus nerve stimulation will help you realise how revolutionary it can be for stress management.

- **Stress Reaction and the Vagus Nerve:**

Stress sets off the sympathetic nervous system, which primes the body for the classic "fight or flight" reaction, which is the body's natural reaction to perceived dangers. To counterbalance the stress reaction and encourage a return to homeostasis, the vagus nerve acts as a relaxing factor.

- **Heart Rate Variability as a Sign of Stress:**

A physiological indicator of the body's capacity to adjust to stress is heart rate variability (HRV), or the fluctuation in the time intervals between heartbeats. Greater vagus nerve activity and improved stress resilience are linked to increased HRV. Higher HRV has been associated with vagus nerve stimulation, which suggests that it may improve the body's stress response systems.

- **Amygdala-influencing factors:**

During periods of prolonged stress, the brain's emotional processing region, the amygdala, is often overactive. The regulation function of the vagus nerve prevents hyperbolic emotional reactions by regulating amygdala activity. A more controlled and adaptable reaction to stresses is facilitated by this modulation.

- **Decrease in Inflammatory Reactions:**

Prolonged stress is intimately linked to inflammation, which is a hidden cause of a number of health problems. It has been shown that vagus nerve stimulation lowers inflammatory reactions, offering a dual advantage by immediately treating stress and lessening the physiological effects of ongoing stress.

- **Methods of Vagus Nerve Stimulation:**

Apart from therapeutic approaches, there are a plethora of methods that enable people to activate their vagus nerve to reduce stress. Practices that activate the vagus nerve, which promotes relaxation and a sensation of peace, include yoga, mindful meditation, and deep breathing exercises.

- **Increasing the Ability to Adapt to New Stressors:**

Physiological resilience is enhanced by vagus nerve stimulation, which makes people more adaptive when faced with stresses in the future. The vagus nerve contributes to long-term mental health by strengthening the parasympathetic response, which protects against the damaging effects of ongoing stress.

- **Integrative Methods for Handling Stress:**

Enhancing vagus nerve function is a common component of holistic methods to stress treatment. Vagus nerve stimulation methods are used in conjunction with lifestyle changes including social relationships, regular physical exercise, and enough sleep to provide a holistic foundation for stress resilience.

- **Vagus nerve functions as a catalyst for mental health.**

The vagus nerve is the conductor of the harmonious interaction between mental and physical health in the complex body's symphony. The vagus nerve plays a vital role in promoting mental health due to its ability to regulate anxiety and sadness as well as its ability to reduce stress.

New avenues for therapeutic treatments are made possible by an understanding of the vagus nerve's effects on neurotransmitter balance, emotional control, and stress response mechanisms. People may promote mental resilience and well-being using a variety of strategies, ranging from accessible everyday routines that stimulate the vagus nerve to therapeutic uses such as vagus nerve stimulation.

It is important to recognize the role the vagus nerve plays in mental health as we manage the complexity of contemporary life. The notion that the body has natural systems for self-healing and self-regulation encourages a paradigm change. Testifying to the complex intelligence woven into our physiological fabric, the vagus nerve provides a means of accessing the transforming potential within, fostering not

just the absence of disease but also the deep
presence of well-being.

Chapter 3

Fighting Inflammation: Revealing the Vital Role of the Vagus Nerve and Reduction Methods

Inflammation is a two-edged sword in the complex dance of the body's physiological reactions. Chronic inflammation may be a silent enemy that contributes to a number of health problems, while being a normal and vital component of the body's defensive processes. We explore the deep connection between inflammation and the vagus nerve in this investigation, elucidating the complex processes at work and shedding light on the useful methods that take use of the vagus nerve's anti-inflammatory properties.

A Key Role for the Vagus Nerve in Inflammation

Long recognized for controlling respiration, heart rate, and digestion, the vagus nerve is now an important link in the complex system that controls inflammation. The body's reaction to an injury or illness is inflammation, which is often characterised by redness, heat, swelling, and discomfort. But when this reaction persists over time, it may lead to a series of health problems, including cardiovascular disease and autoimmune disorders.

- **The Pathway of Cholinergic Anti-Inflammatory Process:**

The cholinergic anti-inflammatory pathway is central to the vagus nerve's function in inflammation. In order to orchestrate a precisely calibrated response to inflammatory signals, this route constitutes an intricate communication network between the neurological system and the immune system.

Acetylcholine is released by the vagus nerve, especially its parasympathetic branch, when the body perceives an inflammatory danger. Immune cells get a soothing signal from this neurotransmitter, telling them to reduce the synthesis of chemicals that promote inflammation. By serving as a conductor in this anti-inflammatory symphony, the vagus nerve contributes to the preservation of a delicate equilibrium and prevents inflammation from intensifying into a harmful, chronic condition.

- **Vagus Nerve and Immune System Control:**

The vagus nerve regulates the immune system in ways that go beyond the body's first reaction to inflammation. Immune cells converse with it in both directions, affecting their activity and encouraging immunological homeostasis. In particular, this regulatory function plays a critical role in avoiding overreactions by the immune system, which may result in autoimmune diseases and chronic inflammation.

- **Influence on the Production of Cytokines:**

An important factor in inflammation is the immune system's signalling molecules, or cytokines. By means of cholinergic transmission, the vagus nerve modulates cytokine synthesis, guaranteeing a modulated and well-regulated immune response. Chronic inflammation is characterised by the unchecked release of pro-inflammatory cytokines, which is inhibited by this complex control.

▪ Reducing Inflammation Using Vagus Nerve Techniques

Equipped with knowledge about the vagus nerve's function in inflammation, we can investigate useful methods to harness this nerve's ability to lower inflammatory reactions. These methods, which have their roots in both traditional wisdom and contemporary science, provide a comprehensive strategy for reducing inflammation and enhancing general health.

▪ Exercises for Deep Breathing:

The foundation of many relaxation techniques, deep breathing exercises, are simple and effective means of activating the vagus nerve. By stimulating the vagus nerve, breathing techniques including diaphragmatic breathing, box breathing, and timed respiration facilitate the release of acetylcholine and start the cholinergic anti-inflammatory pathway.

By contracting the diaphragm, deep, slow breaths cause the brain to produce signals that trigger the parasympathetic nervous system. Acetylcholine, which reduces inflammation and regulates the immunological response, is subsequently released by the vagus nerve in reaction to this. A simple yet powerful method for encouraging vagus nerve activation and lowering chronic inflammation is to include deep breathing into everyday activities.

- **Practices of mindfulness and meditation:**

Meditation and other mindfulness exercises, such as mindful awareness, provide physical advantages for vagus nerve stimulation in addition to mental peace. By triggering the parasympathetic nervous system and increasing vagus nerve activity, mindfulness exercises cultivate a state of calm awareness.

Programs for body scan exercises and mindfulness-based stress reduction (MBSR), which often include meditation, have been demonstrated to be effective in lowering inflammatory markers. These techniques support the vagus nerve's general anti-inflammatory milieu by fostering present-moment awareness and promoting mental calmness.

- **Physical Activity:**
Increased vagus nerve function and decreased inflammation have been associated with regular physical activity,

especially aerobic exercise. Exercises like swimming, cycling, or running improve cardiovascular health and vagal tone, which is a gauge of the activity of the vagus nerve.

The vagus nerve releases acetylcholine in response to aerobic activity, which also alters heart rate and breathing patterns. The anti-inflammatory benefits seen in those who lead busy lifestyles are partly attributed to this release. Including aerobic activity in a regimen is a proactive way to stimulate the vagus nerve, which lowers inflammation and promotes general health.

- **Exposure to cold:**

There has been evidence linking cold exposure—cold air exposure, ice baths, or cold showers—to increased vagus nerve activity. The vagus nerve is involved in a number of adaptation processes that the body uses in reaction to cold.

Being in the cold activates the vagus nerve, which sets off a parasympathetic reaction. Consequently, this enhances the vagus nerve's anti-inflammatory processes. A supplementary tactic for vagus nerve activation and inflammation reduction is regulated and progressive exposure to cold, albeit care should be used, particularly for those with certain health issues.

- **Positive Feelings and Social Links:**

Vagus nerve function is significantly influenced by the calibre of social relationships and happy feelings. Vagal tone is elevated and inflammation is subsequently decreased in response to meaningful social interactions, laughing, and good emotions.

An atmosphere that is hospitable to the vagus nerve is created by doing things that elicit happy feelings, such spending time with loved ones, being grateful, or doing joyful things. Positive emotions and healthy vagus nerve activity are mutually reinforcing, which promotes general wellbeing and lower levels of inflammation.

- **Nutrition & Diet:**

Food decisions may impact inflammation, indirectly influencing the body's general inflammatory state, even if they do not stimulate the vagus nerve directly. The body's innate processes for resolving inflammation are supported by a diet high in omega-3 fatty acids, antioxidants, and anti-inflammatory foods.

Increased vagal tone and decreased inflammation have been linked to omega-3 fatty acids, which are present in walnuts, flaxseeds, and fatty fish. Foods high in antioxidants, such fruits and vegetables, help the body combat oxidative stress, which is connected to inflammation. Keeping an anti-inflammatory diet in check goes hand in hand with promoting vagus nerve activation and general well-being.

Including Vagus Nerve Methods in Holistic Health

Including vagus nerve treatments becomes a complete and powerful strategy in the quest to reduce inflammation and promote overall well-being. A synergistic impact is produced when several vagus nerve stimulation techniques are combined, which improves the body's resilience and capacity to maintain equilibrium.

- **Customised Methods:**

Understanding that wellness habits are personal is crucial. One person's solution may not work the same way for another. Sustained involvement and efficacy are facilitated by comprehending individual preferences, using lifestyle-friendly strategies, and customising activities to meet specific requirements.

- **Integration of the Mind and Body:**
Vagus nerve therapies revolve on the idea of the mind-body link. People may address inflammation reduction from a holistic perspective when they acknowledge the interaction between mental and physical health. Physical and mental-wellness

practices like tai chi and yoga provide a comprehensive way to lower inflammation and stimulate the vagus nerve.

- **Reliability and endurance:**

It takes time and persistence to get noticeable outcomes using vagus nerve methods. These habits have long-term advantages, as with any component of wellbeing. Sustained favourable results are more likely when vagus nerve stimulation treatments are incorporated into a routine and the body is given time to adjust.

The vagus nerve becomes a valuable partner in the fight against inflammation by providing a sophisticated and well-thought-out strategy for immune modulation. After learning about the complex relationship between inflammation and the vagus nerve, people may take an active role in promoting anti-inflammatory responses and improving their general well-being.

People may use the body's innate ability to self-regulate by adopting practices including deep breathing, meditation, cardiovascular activity, exposure to cold, social interaction, and mindful eating. These methods, which have their roots in both traditional knowledge and modern science, provide a comprehensive foundation for lowering inflammation and building resilience.

The wisdom ingrained in vagus nerve procedures becomes more and more pertinent as we traverse the intricacies of contemporary life, where inflammation often hides as a silent contributor to chronic health disorders. It encourages a change in perspective from a reactive to an empowered and proactive attitude to health. With the complex function it plays in regulating inflammation, the vagus nerve extends an invitation to experience holistic wellness—a state in which physical and mental well-being harmonise to produce a symphony of vigour and health.

Chapter 4

Stress Buster: Learning Vagus Nerve Techniques for Relaxation

In today's fast-paced world, stress has become a ubiquitous companion, affecting both mental and physical health. Despite the confusion, the vagus nerve emerges as a powerful ally—a neuronal maestro directing the body's reaction to stress. In this examination, we will look at two crucial vagus nerve techniques: deep breathing exercises and meditation and mindfulness, and how they may help you reduce stress and achieve a sense of calm.

Deep Breathing Exercises: A Symphony of Calm.

- **Understand the Physiology:**

Deep breathing exercises are an old but scientifically validated stress-reduction technique that taps into the intrinsic strength of the vagus nerve. At the heart of this technique is the complex link between the breath and the autonomic nervous system, with the vagus nerve playing a critical role.

Deep, diaphragmatic breathing causes the diaphragm to fall, sending a signal to the brain that activates the parasympathetic nervous system. This, in turn, stimulates the vagus nerve, resulting in the production of acetylcholine—a neurotransmitter that has a soothing effect on the body. The sequence of actions that follows promotes relaxation while counteracting the stress-inducing sympathetic nervous system.

Practical Techniques

- **Diaphragmatic Breath:**
  1. Find a quiet, comfortable place to sit or lay down.
  2. Place one hand on the chest, the other on the abdomen.
  3. Inhale deeply via the nose, allowing the belly to rise while the chest remains relatively motionless.
  4. Exhale gently through pursed lips, feeling the abdomen drop.
  5. Repeat this practice for a few breath cycles, progressively increasing the length of inhalation and exhalation.

- **Box Breathing:**
    1. Inhale deeply through your nose for a count of four.
    2. Hold your breath for a count of four.
    3. Exhale gently through pursed lips for a count of four.
    4. Take a four-count pause at the end of your exhale.
    5. Repeat this rhythmic pattern numerous times, concentrating on a steady and regulated breath.

- **Paced respiration:**
    1. Set a specified breathing rate, such as six breaths per minute.
    2. Maintain a constant beat by inhaling and exhaling for five counts each.
    3. Use a timer or a guided audio resource to help with timed breathing.

4. Allow your breath to flow freely, avoiding forced intake and exhalation.

- **Benefits and Impact on Stress:**

The advantages of deep breathing go beyond the initial sense of tranquillity. Regular use of deep breathing techniques has been linked to:

1. **Cortisol Levels Drop:** Deep breathing has been related to a drop in cortisol, the stress hormone, resulting in a more balanced stress response.

2. **Reduced Heart Rate and Blood Pressure:** Deep breathing activates the vagus nerve, which reduces heart rate and blood pressure, boosting cardiovascular health.

3. Deep breathing promotes awareness and emotional control, helping people to deal with stress more effectively.

4. Deep breathing improves respiratory function by activating the diaphragm and improving respiratory patterns.

Meditation and mindfulness: Nurturing the Vagus Nerve for Serenity.

- **Mind-Body Connection:**

Meditation and mindfulness techniques create a powerful link between the mind and the body, providing a comprehensive approach to stress reduction. These activities, based on ancient traditions and recent science, engage the vagus nerve in a subtle dance of awareness and relaxation.

Mindful Meditation

- **Body Scan Meditation:**
  1. Find a quiet, comfortable place to sit or lay down.
  2. Draw attention to various regions of the body, beginning with the toes and progressing up to the head.
  3. Observe any feelings, tension, or regions of discomfort without passing judgement.
  4. Breathe into each place, allowing a sensation of calm to emerge.
  5. Finish the body scan with a few seconds of total-body awareness.

- **Breath Awareness Meditation:**

    1. Sit comfortably with a straight spine.

    2. Pay attention to the natural flow of the breath, noting each inhalation and exhale.

    3. If your attention wanders, softly refocus it to the breath without judgement.

    4. Develop a feeling of presence and awareness while letting ideas come and go.

- **Loving-kindness Meditation:**

    1. Sit comfortable and shut your eyes.

    2. Begin by offering love and compassion to yourself.

    3. Gradually extend these sentiments to loved ones, acquaintances, and even those with whom you may have disagreements.

4. Cultivate compassion and kindness for all creatures.

5. Finish with a moment of thankfulness and a deep breath.

- **Benefits and Impact on Stress:**

Mindfulness meditation activities have showed a variety of advantages in terms of

stress reduction:

Mindfulness meditation has been associated with enhanced vagal tone, which improves the vagus nerve's regulatory function.

Regular mindfulness practice helps to reduce self-reported stress levels, encouraging a more balanced and resilient reaction to stressors.

- **Improved Emotional Well-Being:**

Mindfulness promotes emotional control,

helping people to handle difficult events more calmly.

- **Improved Cognitive Function:** Meditation activities such as mindfulness have been linked to increased attention, memory, and cognitive flexibility.

- **Altered Brain Structure and Function:** Neuroscientific research suggests that regular meditation may cause changes in brain structure and function, especially in regions associated to stress processing and emotional regulation.

Integrating Vagus Nerve Techniques for Comprehensive Stress Relief

- **Holistic Approach:**

The combination of deep breathing techniques, meditation, and mindfulness gives a comprehensive approach to stress management that addresses both physiological and psychological aspects. Integrating these approaches into regular activities promotes a proactive and powerful approach to stress management.

- **Creating Rituals**

Establishing rituals that include vagus nerve methods improves their efficacy. Whether it's devoting a few minutes each morning to deep breathing or incorporating mindfulness techniques into daily breaks, developing regular routines strengthens the mind-body connection.

- **Adapting to preferences:**

Individual preferences play an important role in maintaining involvement with vagus nerve methods. Exploring numerous versions of deep breathing exercises or trying different meditation approaches helps people to find what works best for their tastes and lifestyle.

- **Mindful Movement Practices:**

Combining vagus nerve procedures with mindful movement activities like yoga or tai chi creates a dynamic approach to stress management. These practices not only include the breath and awareness, but also include modest physical motions that promote total well-being.

Achieving Tranquillity via Vagus Nerve Mastery

In the stress tapestry, the vagus nerve stands out as a soothing force—an sophisticated neurological conductor capable of arranging a quiet symphony. Deep breathing techniques, meditation, and mindfulness practices are the instrumental notes that, when combined, form a melodious journey to stress alleviation and well-being.

Understanding the physiological complexities of vagus nerve activation with these strategies enables people to face stress with fortitude. Whether it's the rhythmic flow of the breath in deep breathing exercises or the contemplative presence developed in mindfulness meditation, each approach urges you to return to the present moment—a place where tension melts away and calm emerges.

As we embrace the skill of mastering vagus nerve methods, we begin on a path of self-realisation and empowerment. This journey is more than just stress management; it's about developing a deep connection with the body's natural ability to be calm and resilient. The vagus nerve is more than simply a biological channel; it is a portal to peace, inviting us to recover our inner refuge in the face of life's pressures.

Chapter 5

The Gut-Brain Connection: Promoting Harmony for Overall Well-Being

The complicated dance of human physiology reveals a remarkable harmony between the gut and the brain, impacting not just digestive health but also general well-being. The vagus nerve is at the centre of this complex connection—a neural highway that connects the stomach and the brain. In this examination, we will look at the vagus nerve's effect on gut health and the larger picture of the gut-brain axis, as well as how it affects our overall well-being.

Gut Health and the Vagus Nerve

- **Anatomy of Vagus Nerve:**

The vagus nerve, sometimes known as the "wandering nerve," extends from the brainstem to numerous organs such as the heart, lungs, and, most importantly, the digestive system. Its complicated branches extend into the digestive system, establishing a dynamic network that coordinates a symphony of communication between the stomach and the brain.

- **Gut-brain communication:**

The vagus nerve functions as a two-way communication route, allowing the stomach and brain to communicate continuously. This bidirectional connection is necessary for digestive system homeostasis and plays an important role in overall gut health.

Regulation of Digestive Processes

The vagus nerve has a significant impact on gut health by regulating critical digestive processes. As food enters the digestive system, the vagus nerve secretes acetylcholine, a neurotransmitter that induces digestion enzyme production and smooth muscle contraction. This orchestration ensures that nutrients are absorbed efficiently and that digestive function is optimum.

- **Modulating gut motility:**

The vagus nerve regulates gut motility by modulating the rhythmic contractions of digestive muscles. Proper motility is essential for moving food through the gastrointestinal system and avoiding problems like constipation or diarrhoea. The vagus nerve's precise regulation helps to coordinate these motions seamlessly, promoting gut health.

The Gut-Brain Axis and Its Effect on Overall Well-being

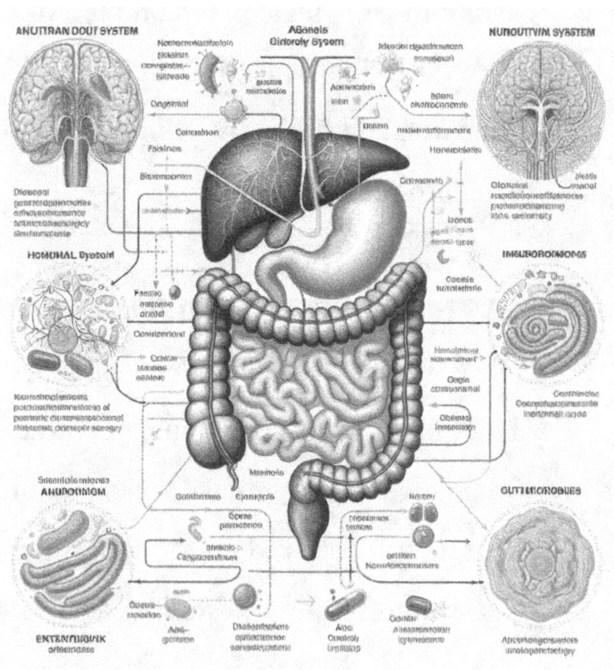

An overview of the gut-brain axis

The gut-brain axis is a complex communication system that incorporates a bidirectional contact between the stomach and brain. This sophisticated network includes not only the vagus nerve, but also hormonal and immunological signals, resulting in a dynamic interaction that goes beyond digestion to affect mental and emotional well-being.

- **Neurotransmitters and Mood Regulation:**

The gut-brain axis is dependent on the generation of neurotransmitters such as serotonin and gamma-aminobutyric acid (GABA). These neurotransmitters, which are often connected with mood regulation, are produced in the stomach and have a considerable impact on emotional states. The vagus nerve, a crucial mediator in this axis, helps to regulate neurotransmitter release.

Impact on Mental and Emotional Well-Being

The gut-brain axis' impact on mental and emotional well-being emphasises the interconnectedness of our physiological and psychological states. This influence has many key features, including:

- **Stress and Cortisol Regulation:**

The gut-brain axis is critical in controlling the stress response, influencing cortisol levels, a hormone intimately associated with stress. The vagus nerve, as a parasympathetic nervous system regulator, inhibits the sympathetic nervous system's activity in response to stress. This balance is vital for avoiding prolonged stress and its negative consequences on mental health.

- **Effects on Anxiety and Depression:**
New study indicates a link between gut health and mental health issues including anxiety and sadness. Dysregulation of the gut-brain axis may lead to neurotransmitter imbalances and inflammatory responses, which may influence mood disorders. The vagus nerve's regulatory function becomes critical in maintaining balance along this axis.

- **Role in neurologic conditions:**
The gut-brain axis has consequences beyond mood disorders, including neurological illnesses like Parkinson's and Alzheimer's. The vagus nerve allows communication

between the stomach and the brain, which may impact the evolution of various disorders. There is continuing research into therapies that target the gut-brain axis for neuroprotection.

Strategies for Developing a Healthy Gut-Brain Connection

Understanding the importance of the gut-brain link offers up possibilities for cultivating a healthy interaction between these two critical systems. Strategies for supporting a healthy gut-brain axis include:

- **Dietary Considerations:**

A well-balanced and diversified diet is important for gut health and the gut-brain axis. Fibre-rich meals, fermented foods, and prebiotics nurture the gut bacteria, creating a positive environment for general health. The vagus nerve, affected by dietary variables, reacts to signals from a healthy gut.

- **Probiotics and the gut microbiota:**

Probiotics are living microorganisms with possible health benefits that help to balance the intestinal flora. According to research, some probiotics may have a favourable effect on the gut-brain axis, altering neurotransmitter synthesis and immunological responses. The makeup of the microbiota influences the vagus nerve's communication with the gut, stressing the need of probiotics in promoting gut health.

- **Stress-Management Techniques:**

Given the effects of stress on the gut-brain axis, stress management practices are essential for general well-being. Mindfulness meditation, deep breathing exercises, and yoga all engage the vagus nerve and contribute to a healthy stress response. These strategies promote resilience and the smooth operation of the gut-brain axis.

- **Regular physical activity:**

Exercise has been demonstrated to change the makeup of the gut bacteria and improve communication between the gut and brain. Regular physical exercise promotes intestinal health, reduces inflammation, and improves mood management. The vagus nerve, which is engaged during exercise, adds to the overall effect on the gut-brain link.

- **Quality sleep:**

Sleep is essential for general health, and it affects the gut-brain axis. Adequate and high-quality sleep promotes intestinal health by allowing for healing and regeneration. Sleep disruptions may have an influence on the gut microbiota and lead to abnormalities in the gut-brain axis. Prioritising good sleep habits improves communication between the stomach and the brain.

Developing Synergy for Holistic Well-Being

In the complicated story of human health, the gut-brain link, aided by the vagus nerve's nuanced effect, emerges as a key participant. Understanding the complexities of this relationship reveals more than just its involvement in digestion; it also reveals a fundamental interaction that defines our mental, emotional, and general health.

Nurturing a healthy gut-brain axis requires a multimodal strategy that includes food awareness, stress management strategies, physical exercise, and prioritising excellent sleep. In this comprehensive attempt, the vagus nerve serves as a conductor, arranging a harmonic symphony between the stomach and the brain.

As we explore into the realms of gut health and physical system interconnection, we discover not just a narrative of digestion, but also a story of synergy—a narrative in which the well-being of the stomach impacts the well-being of the mind and vice versa. By fostering this synergy, we begin on a path toward holistic health, where the gut-brain connection becomes a source of resilience, balance, and long-term well-being.

Chapter 6

Unleashing the Healing Power Within: The Role of the Vagus Nerve in Self-Healing

The vagus nerve is an often-overlooked yet powerful factor for healing inside the human body. Emerging science and traditional knowledge combine to reveal the vagus nerve's fundamental significance in facilitating self-healing, allowing us to tap into our inner talents. In this investigation, we will look at the processes of vagus nerve stimulation and the critical function it plays in releasing the healing force that exists inside each human.

Innate Healing Abilities Within Us

▪ Understanding Your Body's Innate Wisdom:

Our bodies have a complex intelligence, a self-regulating mechanism that strives for balance and well-being. This innate intelligence orchestrates a symphony of physiological processes designed to preserve balance. From the molecular level to the delicate dance of neurotransmitters, the body's intrinsic powers for repair and rejuvenation are built into the very fabric of our existence.

▪ Holistic Approach to Healing:

True healing goes beyond the absence of sickness. It takes a comprehensive approach to well-being, including physical, mental, and emotional elements. The intrinsic healing skills inside us react to diverse stimuli, and the vagus nerve is an important conductor in this self-healing symphony.

Utilising the Potential of Vagus Nerve Stimulation

- **Understanding Vagus Nerve Stimulation.**

The vagus nerve is a long, wandering cranial nerve that plays an important role in the body's autonomic nervous system. The vagus nerve, which has long been known for its function in controlling heart rhythm and digestion, has now emerged as an important factor in self-healing. Vagus nerve stimulation entails deliberate actions that activate and engage this brain system, resulting in a cascade of responses that enhance well-being.

▪ Effects on the Parasympathetic Nervous System:

The effect of vagus nerve stimulation on the parasympathetic nervous system (PNS) is crucial to its operation. The PNS, sometimes known as the "rest and digest" system, helps to balance the sympathetic nervous system's stress-inducing effects. Vagus nerve stimulation stimulates the PNS, resulting in relaxation, restoration, and improved self-healing abilities.

▪ Acetylcholine Release

The capacity of vagus nerve stimulation to produce acetylcholine, a neurotransmitter with significant effects on the body, is what makes it so effective. Acetylcholine works as a relaxing and anti-inflammatory agent, impacting a variety of physiological processes. Acetylcholine release, which modulates immune responses and regulates inflammation, sets the setting for the body's intrinsic healing mechanisms to take effect.

- **Cholinergic Anti-inflammatory Pathway:**

The cholinergic anti-inflammatory pathway is an important mechanism used by the vagus nerve to promote self-healing. This complex network includes the release of acetylcholine, which suppresses the formation of pro-inflammatory chemicals. The vagus nerve promotes healing by decreasing the inflammatory response, both in acute and chronic diseases.

The Vagus Nerve and Self-Healing

- **Modulating the immune response:**

The vagus nerve carefully tunes the immune system, which serves as a sentinel against intruders as well as a facilitator of recovery. The vagus nerve controls the immune response by communicating with immune cells, avoiding undue inflammation and fostering a balanced response to threats. This immunological regulation is a key component of the vagus nerve's self-healing function.

- **Promoting Neuroplasticity:**

The vagus nerve influences neuroplasticity, which is the capacity of the brain to restructure and generate new neural connections. The vagus nerve helps the nervous system adapt by communicating with the brain via an extensive network. This flexibility is essential for learning, memory, and the resilience needed for self-healing.

Balancing the Autonomic Nervous System.

The autonomic nervous system, which includes sympathetic and parasympathetic branches, is critical in the body's reaction to stress and relaxation. The vagus nerve functions as a regulator, regulating the autonomic nervous system and ensuring that the body's resources are properly distributed. This equilibrium is essential for healthy physiological function and self-healing.

- **Influence on Emotional Well-Being**

Beyond its physiological function, the vagus nerve has a significant effect on mental well-being. The vagus nerve, which acts as a conduit between the stomach and the brain, helps to regulate mood and stress. The vagus nerve promotes emotional equilibrium, which generates a mental environment favourable to the self-healing process.

Practical Ways to Use Vagus Nerve Stimulation:

- **Deep Breathing Exercises:**
Deep breathing techniques, such as diaphragmatic breathing, engage the vagus nerve and promote acetylcholine release. Incorporating deep breathing into everyday activities is a simple yet effective method for fostering self-healing.

- **Meditation and mindfulness practices:**

Mindfulness meditation, with its emphasis on the present moment and breath awareness, stimulates the vagus nerve. Regular practice promotes relaxation and boosts the body's natural healing abilities.

- **Aerobic Exercise:**

Regular aerobic exercise not only benefits general health, but it also improves vagal tone—a measure of the vagus nerve's activity. This increased vagal tone helps the body's resistance and self-healing powers.

- **Social connections:**

Positive social contacts and meaningful relationships enhance vagus nerve function. Nurturing social relationships produces an atmosphere that promotes emotional well-being and self-healing.

- **Cold Exposure**

Controlled cold exposure, such cold showers or ice baths, activates the vagus nerve. When undertaken with prudence, this technique promotes self-healing by activating the parasympathetic nervous system.

Promoting a Self-Healing Lifestyle:

- **Mind-Body Integration:**

Recognizing the interdependence of the mind and body is a fundamental component in developing a self-healing lifestyle. Yoga and tai chi are examples of practices that combine mental and physical well-being. They provide a holistic approach that is consistent with the regulating function of the vagus nerve.

- **Nutrition and gut health:**

A balanced and nutritious diet that promotes intestinal health helps to stimulate the vagus nerve. Probiotic-rich diets, fibre, and anti-inflammatory substances promote internal healing.

- **Quality sleep:**

Prioritising excellent sleep enables the body to participate in restorative processes. The vagus nerve, which is stimulated during sleep, helps to the body's self-healing capabilities, underlining the need for a consistent sleep schedule.

empowering the journey of self-healing.

In the symphony of the body's natural intelligence, the vagus nerve serves as a conductor, arranging the songs of self-heal. Individuals may release their healing potential by learning and actively engaging the mechanics of vagus nerve stimulation. The vagus nerve creates a narrative of resilience and vigour by modifying immunological responses and impacting emotional well-being.

As we begin on our road of self-healing, let us acknowledge the collaboration between contemporary ideas and old wisdom. The vagus nerve encourages us to create habits that correspond with our bodies' intrinsic abilities, encouraging a lifestyle in which self-healing becomes a natural and powerful expression of well-being. This inquiry reveals not just the possibility for healing, but also a deep affirmation of our body's power to grow, renew, and flourish from within.

Chapter 7

Practical Tips for Daily Life: Promoting a Vagus Nerve-Friendly Lifestyle

In today's fast-paced world, when stress and expectations sometimes take precedence, creating a lifestyle that supports the vagus nerve becomes critical. The vagus nerve, a crucial participant in the autonomic nervous system, controls our body's relaxation response and self-healing capabilities. In this research, we will discover practical techniques for effortlessly integrating vagus nerve workouts into everyday routines and building a lifestyle that aligns with the intrinsic knowledge of this neurological conductor.

Understanding the Vagus Nerve's Role in Daily Well-Being

Overview of the Vagus Nerve:

The vagus nerve, named after the Latin word for "wandering," certainly lives true to its name. This cranial nerve runs from the brainstem down the body, branching into numerous organs such as the heart, lungs, and digestive system. Its widespread effect puts the vagus nerve as a major regulator of the autonomic nervous system, which is in charge of involuntary body activities.

Balancing the Autonomic Nervous System.

The vagus nerve's purpose is around its impact on the autonomic nervous system (ANS), which includes the sympathetic and parasympathetic branches. While the sympathetic system prepares us for the well-known "fight or flight" reaction, the parasympathetic system, guided by the vagus nerve, ushers in the "rest and digest" state. Balancing these systems is critical for everyday wellness, stress management, and overall health.

Integrating Vagus Nerve Exercises into Daily Routines

- **Deep Breathing Exercises:**

1. **Diaphragmatic Breathing:** Locate a quiet area, sit or lay down, and put a hand on your abdomen. Inhale deeply through the nose, allowing the belly to rise, then exhale slowly through pursed lips, feeling the abdomen sink. Repeat the repetitive pattern for a few

minutes to stimulate the vagus nerve and promote relaxation.

2. **Box Breathing:** Inhale, hold, exhale, and pause for a count of four. This systematic breathing technique not only relaxes the mind but also stimulates the vagus nerve, which promotes balance.

- **Mindfulness meditation:**

1. **Body Scan Meditation:** Set out a few minutes every day to practise body scan meditation. Concentrate on each area of the body, from toes to head, developing awareness and relaxation. Mindfulness meditation activates the vagus nerve, causing a sensation of calm.

2. **Loving-Kindness Meditation:** Extend your sentiments of love and compassion to yourself and others. This technique not only improves emotional well-being but also activates the vagus nerve, resulting in a happy attitude.

- **Aerobic Exercise:**

1. **Daily Walks or Runs:** Participate in aerobic exercises such as walking or running. The rhythmic exercise and increased heart rate not only improve cardiovascular health, but they also raise vagal tone, which helps the vagus nerve function.

2. Make exercising more pleasant by including dance or cardio routines into your program. The combination

of activity and higher heart rate activates the vagus nerve, which improves general well-being.

- **Social connections:**

1. Prioritise social ties and devote quality time to loved ones. Positive interactions and laughing stimulate the vagus nerve, which increases emotional resilience.

2. **Express thanks:** Make it a regular practice to express your thanks. Acknowledging the good parts of life, whether via writing or vocal affirmations, stimulates the vagus nerve and enhances overall well-being.

Developing a Vagus Nerve-Friendly Lifestyle

Mindful nutrition

- **Embrace a Balanced Diet:** Eat entire, nutrient-dense foods that promote intestinal health. A varied and healthy diet promotes the gut-brain connection, which is linked to the vagus nerve.

Include probiotic-rich foods, such as yoghurt, kefir, and fermented vegetables. Promoting a healthy gut microbiome improves vagus nerve function.

Quality sleep:

- **Establish a Sleep Routine:** Make a regular sleep schedule by going to bed and getting up at the same time every day.

Quality sleep is necessary for vagus nerve activity and general health.

- **Create a Relaxing Bedtime Ritual:** Before going to bed, do something relaxing like read, stretch gently, or do deep breathing exercises. This tells the vagus nerve that it's time to rest and relax.

Hydration and cold exposure:

- **Stay Hydrated:** Proper hydration improves general health, including vagus nerve function. Make sure you drink enough water throughout the day.

- **Cold Showers or Cold Water Immersion:** Try regulated cold exposure, such as cold showers or immersion in cold water. Cold exposure activates the vagus nerve, which may revitalise the neural system.

Mind and Body Practices:

▪ **Yoga or Tai Chi:** Incorporate mind-body exercises like yoga or tai chi into your regimen. These techniques not only activate the vagus nerve, but also promote awareness and physical well-being.

Take small pauses throughout the day to practise mindful breathing. Whether at your desk or in a quiet corner, a few minutes of concentrated breathing may help to reset the nervous system and increase vagus nerve activity.

Developing Consistency and Mindful Presence

Incorporating vagus nerve exercises into everyday life does not imply following a rigorous plan, but rather building a lifestyle based on consistency and attentive presence. Below are a few guiding principles:

- **Consistency:** Make these techniques a daily part of your routine. Consistency is essential for maximising the advantages of vagus nerve stimulation.

- **Adapt to Your Preferences:** Try various workouts and see what works for you. Customise your schedule to meet your needs while guaranteeing sustainability.

- **Mindful Integration:** Instead of considering these exercises as extra duties, incorporate them carefully into your regular habits. This may be a quick meditation during a break, or a mindful breathing practice before meals.

- **Listen to Your Body:** Be aware of how your body reacts. The objective is to have a great and long-lasting experience, so listen to your body and make adjustments as required.

Chapter 8

Enhancing Wholeness and Wellness: A Symphony of Holistic Well-Being

In the complex dance of life, real well-being goes beyond the absence of sickness. It entails a harmonic combination of mental, emotional, and physical well-being—a condition in which the symphony of our life vibrates with harmony and vigour. The vagus nerve is central to this symphony, a brain conductor that, when activated consciously, serves as a guiding force in the quest of comprehensive well-being. In this inquiry, we will look at the art of enhancing wholeness and wellbeing by including vagus nerve treatments and cultivating balance across all aspects of our being.

The Vagus Nerve as a Pathway to Wholeness

- **Understanding the Vagus Nerve's Multiple Roles:**

The vagus nerve, frequently referred to as the body's communication superhighway, weaves a complex network throughout the body, linking the brain with other organs. Its importance goes well beyond controlling physiological activities; it acts as a link between mental, emotional, and physical health. Understanding the vagus nerve's various contributions is critical while embarking on a path of completeness.

Integrating Vagus Nerve Techniques for Holistic Wellness:

Embracing Mind-Body Practices

- **Yoga for Mind-Body Integration:** Yoga, with its focus on breath control, mindful movement, and meditation, stimulates the vagus nerve. Yoga, via its different positions and careful breathing, serves as a conduit for linking the mind and body, supporting overall health.

- **Tai Chi for Flowing Harmony:** Tai Chi is a gentle and flowing martial art that provides contemplative movement experiences. Its rhythmic patterns stimulate the vagus nerve, causing relaxation and a sensation of harmony. The combination of breath and movement results in a dance of totality.

Music and sound therapy

- **Harmonizing Vibrations:** Music, particularly when created for therapeutic purposes, has the ability to alter the vagus nerve. Certain frequencies and rhythms may activate the vagus nerve, resulting in a resonance that promotes relaxation and overall well-being. Sound therapy emerges as a novel method for enhancing overall health.

- **Guided Vagus Nerve Meditations:** Meditation techniques designed to stimulate the vagus nerve provide a direct path to overall well-being. These guided meditations emphasise breath awareness, positive affirmations, and purposeful relaxation to foster a balanced mental and emotional state.

Expressive Arts and Creativity

- **Art & Creativity for Emotional Release:** Expressive arts, such as painting, writing, and other creative activities, give an avenue for emotional expression. The vagus nerve, which is closely tied to the brain's emotional centres, reacts to creative pursuits by encouraging emotional release and balance.

- **Laughter therapy:** As the saying goes, laughter is the best medicine. Genuine and uncontrolled laughing activates the vagus nerve, causing a cascade of good physiological effects. Integrating laughter into everyday life becomes a joyous discipline in the search of wholeness.

Creating Balance in Mental, Emotional, and Physical Health

Emotional Resilience and Vagus Nerve Harmony.

The vagus nerve plays a critical role in the complex link between emotions and well-being. Individuals may increase their sense of completeness and wellbeing by cultivating emotional resilience. Techniques for improving emotional balance include:

- **Mindful Awareness activities:** Mindfulness activities promote present-moment awareness, which corresponds to the vagus nerve's function in regulating emotional reactions. attentive breathing, body scans, and attentive observation serve as a basis for emotional balance.

- **thankfulness as a Positive Emotion:** Aside from its psychological effects, the practice of thankfulness stimulates the vagus nerve. Expressing appreciation triggers pleasant feelings, which contribute to a healthy emotional landscape and general well-being.

- **Physical health and vagus nerve activation:**
Physical well-being is inextricably linked to vagus nerve function. The vagus nerve is important for both cardiovascular health and immunological function. Techniques that promote physical health and general wellbeing include:

Aerobic exercise increases the cardiovascular system while also improving vagal tone. The subsequent increase in vagus nerve activity adds to a general sensation of well-being.

- **Nutrition to Promote Gut-Brain Harmony:** A well-balanced and nutritious diet supports the gut-brain connection, which is inextricably related to the vagus nerve. Prioritising whole meals, which are high in nutrients and promote gastrointestinal health, produces an environment that encourages vagus nerve activity.

Harmonizing Dimensions of Well-Being:

Mind-Emotion-Body Synergy

Mind, emotion, and body work together to create wholeness and wellbeing. The vagus nerve, with its far-reaching effects, serves as a unifying factor in this symphony. Techniques that facilitate the integration of these aspects include:

- **Mind-Body Practices:** Yoga, tai chi, and meditation integrate the mental, emotional, and physical components of well-being. These practices bring the aspects of self together via deliberate movement, breath awareness, and mindfulness.

Emotional intelligence is built on the understanding and regulation of emotions. The vagus nerve, which is intricately related to emotional centres, reacts to emotional awareness and control, helping to maintain balance.

- **Holistic Lifestyle Choices:** Adopting a lifestyle that recognizes the interdependence of mind, emotion, and body is crucial. From great sleep to thoughtful diet, each decision adds a note to the symphony of well-being, guided by the vagus nerve.

Cultivating Wholeness is a Lifelong Journey.

The search for completeness and wellbeing is a lifetime adventure, with the vagus nerve acting as a guiding compass. As people explore the domains of thought, emotion, and body, they are encouraged to:

- **Embrace Curiosity:** Approach the trip with curiosity and openness. Investigate several vagus nerve procedures to see what resonates particularly with your tastes.

- **Celebrate Progress:** Recognize and celebrate little accomplishments along the road. Whether it's a moment of emotional equilibrium or a commitment to regular exercise, each step adds to the symphony of well-being.

- **Listen to Your Body's Wisdom:** The body expresses its demands and answers. Pay close attention to the body's indications, and alter your routines and decisions appropriately.

- **Connect with the Community:** Share your journey with others who share your values. Whether via support groups, wellness communities, or social

connections, collaborative discovery
enriches the holistic well-being journey.

Chapter 9

Success Stories: Overcome Adversity with Vagus Nerve Practices.

In the fabric of personal well-being, success tales serve as beacons of inspiration, illuminating the transformational potential of vagus nerve therapies. Individuals have not only battled, but also won over, the shadows of anxiety, sadness, and stress. These success stories are more than just testimonials; they are deep journeys of perseverance, self-discovery, and an unyielding determination to live a life of energy and completeness.

Exploring the Path to Transformation:

From Darkness to Light: A Journey Through Anxiety.

Introducing Sarah, a young worker navigating the turbulent seas of anxiety. The incessant onslaught of anxieties and the overpowering grip of dread had thrown a pall over her everyday existence. Sarah sought sanctuary and discovered the amazing influence of vagus nerve activities.

Adding deep breathing techniques to her program became a lifeline. Sarah engaged her vagus nerve with each purposeful breath, which set off a chain reaction of relaxing benefits. Anxiety eased its grip gradually but steadily. Sarah's path from darkness to light was not quick, but her consistent vagus nerve practices served as a compass, leading her to tranquillity.

Breaking the Chains of Depression

James' narrative emerges as a moving examination of victory over the bonds of despair. Faced with the crushing weight of sorrow, James found peace in the soft embrace of vagus nerve stimulation. Mindful meditation and loving-kindness activities become an essential component of his daily regimen.

As James entered the worlds of his emotions, the vagus nerve reacted with a gentle dance of healing. The production of positive neurotransmitters and the modification of his emotional reactions signalled a turning point. James' success story demonstrates the transforming impact of vagus nerve activities in removing the veil of sadness and bringing a fresh feeling of optimism.

Inspiration Amidst the Struggles

Resilience under Chronic Stress:
Emma's journey takes place against the background of chronic stress, a constant force that threatens to destroy the fabric of her well-being. Her daily life had become a fight, and the impact on her emotional and physical health was obvious. Emma found resilience contained inside the vagus nerve while navigating the stress labyrinth.

Emma's stress-reduction arsenal included vagus nerve tactics like guided meditations and mindful breathing pauses. When stimulated, the vagus nerve arranged a symphony of calm, counteracting the negative consequences of persistent stress. Emma's tale demonstrates the strength of the human spirit and the importance of vagus nerve activities in fostering resilience.

Finding Light beyond the Shadows

Mark's story is about discovering light beyond the shadows of worry and tension. The demands of a high-pressure work have had a negative impact on his mental health. Mark sought a comprehensive approach and accepted the transforming power of vagus nerve methods.

Mark developed self-care habits that included daily walks and mindful deep breathing. The vagus nerve reacted by regulating his autonomic nervous system, resulting in a sensation of balance. Mark's success story serves as a reminder that, among the hustle and bustle of life, the vagus nerve acts as a guiding force, providing a route to light even in the darkest of times.

A Tapestry of Well-being Woven Using Vagus Nerve Practices

- **Connecting the Mind, Body, and Spirit:** These success tales all have one thing in common: a deep connection between mind, body, and soul. Vagus nerve activities operate as the loom, creating this rich tapestry of well-being. Sarah, James, Emma, and Mark's success stories demonstrate the vagus nerve's ability to enable a comprehensive metamorphosis.

- **Empowerment via Self-Healing:**

The central theme of these tales is empowerment via self-healing. The vagus nerve, frequently referred to as the body's internal peacemaker, serves as a catalyst for people to retake control over their own health. Success stories are about more than simply overcoming obstacles; they represent a journey of self-discovery, tenacity, and each person's intrinsic ability to heal.

Inspiring Others on their Journey

- **Creating a Community of Support:**

Beyond individual accomplishments, these success tales spread, motivating others on similar paths. Sarah, James, Emma, and

Mark work together to construct a community—one in which the transforming potential of vagus nerve practices is shared, appreciated, and accepted.

- **Encourage a Mindset of Possibility:**

Success tales inspire a sense of potential. They undermine the narrative of powerlessness that is often connected with mental health issues. By sharing victory stories, these tales become beacons of hope, urging others to investigate the possibilities of vagus nerve activities and begin on their pathways to well-being.

Chapter 10

Identifying Potential Pitfalls and Misconceptions About Vagus Nerve Stimulation

As interest in vagus nerve stimulation develops, so does the demand for clarity in the middle of a plethora of information. While the potential advantages are enticing, there are several frequent hazards and myths that should be investigated. This conversation tries to shed light on these complexities, giving a compass for anyone navigating the world of vagus nerve stimulation.

Pitfall: Oversimplification of Vagus Nerve Stimulation

Oversimplifying vagus nerve stimulation is a typical problem. The vagus nerve is a complicated structure that is closely linked to many biological systems. Oversimplifying its stimulation may result in excessive expectations and a misunderstanding of the many processes involved.

- **Addressing Concerns: Emphasising Multiple Effects:**

It's critical to understand that vagus nerve stimulation affects not just mental well-being, but also physiological processes including heart rate, digestion, and inflammation. Addressing concerns entails stressing the various impacts of vagus nerve stimulation and promoting a comprehensive awareness of its role in overall health.

Clearing Up Misconceptions

- **Misconception:Instant Results:**

The expectation of immediate outcomes is a frequent misperception. While some people may see instant advantages, the transformational impacts of vagus nerve stimulation are usually delayed. Clarifying this myth fosters patience and a realistic outlook on the timescale for favourable results.

- **Concerns: Setting Realistic Expectations**

Setting reasonable expectations is critical for dealing with time difficulties. Individuals starting vagus nerve stimulation should be aware that the time it takes to see substantial results may vary. Educating people about the process's progressive nature encourages them to be more educated and patient.

Misconception: A "one-size-fits-all" approach

Another myth is that vagus nerve stimulation is a one-size-fits-all treatment. Individuals react differently to different tactics, so what works for one person may not work for another. To clear up this misperception, promote a customised strategy to vagus nerve stimulation that is suited to individual preferences and requirements.

- **Addressing Concerns: Promoting Exploration and Adaptation.**

To address concerns about individual variations, it is critical to foster inquiry and adaptability. Individuals should feel liberated to experiment with a range of vagus nerve stimulation treatments rather than being forced to stick to a single approach. This technique enables the discovery of strategies that are particularly appealing to each individual.

Pitfalls in Technique Application

- **Pitfall: Misapplication of Techniques:** Misunderstanding or improper administration of vagus nerve stimulation methods may be a serious mistake. Mistakes in application, whether via inappropriate breathing exercises or inconsistent practice, might reduce the efficacy of stimulation.

- **Addressing Concerns: Setting Clear Guidelines and Supervision**:

Addressing concerns about method implementation requires explicit standards and, in certain situations, supervised teaching. Guided meditation sessions, educational films, and working with competent specialists may all help you comprehend and use vagus nerve stimulation procedures more effectively.

Misconceptions about Invasiveness

- **Misconception: Invasive Procedures only:**

A common misperception is that vagus nerve stimulation is exclusively used in invasive medical operations. While medicinal therapies are available, non-invasive methods such as breathing exercises, meditation, and lifestyle modifications may successfully activate the vagus nerve.

▪ Addressing Concerns: Highlighting Non-invasive Alternatives:

To address concerns about invasiveness, it is critical to show the variety of non-invasive options. Individuals should be aware that integrating vagus nerve stimulation into their everyday lives may be as easy as practising mindfulness and making lifestyle changes, making it more accessible to a wider range of people.

Pitfalls in Expectations Management

▪ Pitfall: Reliance on Vagus Nerve Stimulation Alone

One possible drawback is relying only on vagus nerve stimulation to address complicated health issues. While it may be an important component of well-being, expecting it to solve all problems on its own may leave you disappointed.

▪ Addressing Concerns with Complementary Approaches:

To address dependence issues, it is critical to stress the importance of vagus nerve stimulation as part of a comprehensive strategy. Encouraging people to combine it with other well-established practices like regular exercise, a healthy diet, and professional healthcare results in a more holistic well-being plan.

Misconceptions of Perceived Risk

- **Misconception: Perceived risk of negative effects:**

Individuals may be hesitant to try vagus nerve stimulation due to perceived dangers, such as worries about possible side effects. While major adverse effects are uncommon, overcoming this misunderstanding requires presenting precise information about the safety profile of various stimulation modalities.

- **Addressing concerns: Communicating safety and risk factors:**

Addressing perceived risk concerns requires open communication regarding the safety and possible risks of vagus nerve stimulation. Individuals should have access to balanced information that allows them to make educated choices, creating trust in the profession.

▪ Understanding the Details of Vagus Nerve Stimulation

Navigating possible traps and misunderstandings in the rapidly evolving world of vagus nerve stimulation is critical for enabling informed involvement. Individuals may approach vagus nerve stimulation with a nuanced viewpoint if they grasp the diverse nature of the therapy, clear any misunderstandings, and address any concerns.

As we navigate the complexities of well-being, the journey with vagus nerve stimulation becomes a dynamic exploration—one in which individuals are empowered with knowledge, encouraged to adapt practices to their specific needs, and given a realistic understanding of the transformative process.

In the symphony of well-being, vagus nerve stimulation plays a melody of possibility, providing people with a route to improved health and vitality. Navigating the intricacies enables us to appreciate the rich tapestry of possibilities within the world of vagus nerve stimulation—a tapestry woven with threads of clarity, comprehension, and the promise of overall well-being.

Chapter 11

Unveiling the Scientific Basis of Vagus Nerve Stimulation: A Symphony of Research and Expert Perspectives

In the area of holistic well-being, the symphony of science resonates with deep harmony—the scientific basis of vagus nerve stimulation emerges as a lyrical study. The transformational potential of stimulating the vagus nerve becomes clearer as we dig into research papers and seek expert opinions. This debate tries to peel back the layers of data supporting vagus nerve stimulation's effectiveness, allowing for a more in-depth knowledge of its effects on mental, emotional, and physical well-being.

Rhythm of Research Studies

- **Melodic Notes of Validation**

Numerous studies have validated the effectiveness of vagus nerve stimulation. A symphony of data has developed, confirming the several advantages of activating this important brain circuit. From mental health to inflammatory control, the scientific environment is brimming with studies that add to the chorus of knowledge.

- **Harmony in Mental Health.**

Research in the field of mental health supports the usefulness of vagus nerve stimulation. Studies have looked at its involvement in anxiety and depression management, and the results indicate that it has a substantial influence on mood control. The cyclic dance of neurotransmitters induced by vagus nerve stimulation becomes an effective ally in the symphony of emotional well-being.

- **Resonance in Stress Reduction:**

The effect of vagus nerve stimulation on stress relief has been a focus of scientific research. Studies look at the complex interaction between the vagus nerve and the autonomic nervous system, with a focus on its involvement in controlling the stress response. The harmonic cadence produced by vagus nerve activity seems to be a possible cure to chronic stress.

- **Counterpoint in Inflammation Management:**

The field of inflammation control serves as a counterweight to the symphony. The vagus nerve is linked to inflammatory processes, and research shows that it has the capacity to reduce inflammation. As the vagus nerve performs its symphony, it orchestrates an anti-inflammatory response, providing a soothing melody for patients suffering from inflammatory disorders.

Experts' viewpoints

- **Voices of authority in the orchestra:**
Experts offer their authoritative voices to the scientific symphony, amplifying the relevance of vagus nerve stimulation. These specialists, ranging from neuroscientists to healthcare professionals, provide various opinions on the effects of vagus nerve stimulation.

- **Dr. Elena Rodriguez, neuroscientist**

Dr. Elena Rodriguez, a renowned neuroscientist, highlights the neurobiological basis for vagus nerve stimulation. Her study sheds light on the complicated connections between the vagus nerve and the brain, revealing the methods by which stimulation affects cognitive functioning. According to her, the symphony of vagus nerve activity goes beyond emotional well-being to cognitive improvement.

- **Dr. Maya Patel is a clinical psychologist.**

Dr. Maya Patel, a seasoned clinical psychologist, adds a therapeutic perspective to vagus nerve stimulation. Drawing on her professional expertise, she describes the transforming implications of combining vagus nerve methods into mental health treatment strategies. In her opinion, the symphony becomes a therapeutic modality, providing people with a unique channel for their healing journeys.

- **Professor Jonathan Turner, cardiologist:**

Prof. Jonathan Turner discusses the cardiovascular ramifications of vagus nerve stimulation from a cardiological standpoint. His study emphasises the importance of the vagus nerve in heart rate regulation and cardiovascular health. Prof. Turner believes that the symphony of vagus nerve activity contributes not only to emotional and mental well-being, but also to cardiovascular system harmony.

- **Dr. Linda Simmons, immunologist**

Dr. Linda Simmons brings her immunology knowledge to the symphony, focusing on the immunomodulatory effects of vagus nerve stimulation. Her study focuses on the communication network between the vagus nerve and the immune system, revealing how vagus nerve methods might alter immunological responses. She sees the symphony as a conductor of immunological harmony.

Integrating insights:

- **Harmonising Diverse Perspectives:**
The incorporation of findings from neuroscientists, clinical psychologists, cardiologists, and immunologists results in a harmonious tapestry of comprehension. The symphony of vagus nerve stimulation, as seen through the eyes of these specialists, goes beyond a single note and becomes a symphonic composition that resonates with the nuances of the mind-body link.

- **Linking the Mind, Emotion, and Body:** Experts agree that the symphony of vagus nerve stimulation involves a delicate connection between thought, emotion, and body. The neuronal connections travelled by the vagus nerve serve as a bridge, enabling the symphony to balance mental and emotional well-being and physiological functions. This interconnectivity becomes a central motif in the story of vagus nerve activity.

Chapter 12

Harmony in Healing: Incorporating Vagus Nerve Techniques into Modern Medicine

In the changing landscape of healthcare, a harmonic blending of conventional and alternative techniques is taking place—a symphony in which the vagus nerve takes centre stage. As we investigate the integration of vagus nerve methods into conventional medicine, a story of partnership and optimum healing emerges. This debate digs into the harmony of contemporary medicine and ancient knowledge encompassed in vagus nerve therapies, resulting in a song of holistic well-being.

The Vagus Nerve As A Healing Conductor

- **Understanding The Vagus Nerve's Role in Health:**

The integration is based on a thorough knowledge of the vagus nerve's function in health. Beyond its historical importance in traditional therapeutic techniques, contemporary science acknowledges the vagus nerve as a brain conductor that orchestrates a symphony of reactions, from emotional control to immunological modulation. This realisation serves as the basis for incorporating vagus nerve methods into the fabric of conventional treatment.

- **From ancient wisdom to modern applications:**

The integration process starts with the recognition of ancient knowledge encoded in vagus nerve procedures. Deep breathing, meditation, and mindfulness are ancient therapeutic practices that find resonance in contemporary medicine. The transition is more than simply a return to old methods; it is also an acknowledgment of their ongoing significance in managing the complexity of today's health concerns.

Integrating Vagus Nerve Techniques into Mainstream Healthcare

- **Mental Health as a focal point:**

Mental health is one of the key areas of integration. As the incidence of anxiety and depression increases, conventional healthcare is embracing vagus nerve therapies as supplementary modalities. Mindfulness-based techniques, such as guided meditation and deep breathing exercises, have become standard components of mental health treatment strategies.

- **Stress Management in Clinical Setting:**

In therapeutic settings, stress management is a critical use for vagus nerve methods. Healthcare practitioners understand the effect of chronic stress on general health and use techniques such as biofeedback and progressive muscle relaxation, both of which correspond to vagus nerve activity. The integration goes beyond medications, focusing on self-care activities that help people manage their pressures.

- **Cardiology and Vagal Tone Enhancement**

Within cardiology, there is a partnership between vagus nerve procedures and heart health. Interventions are aimed at improving vagal tone, which is a measure of the vagus nerve's activity. Aerobic exercise, which has been shown to improve vagal tone, is suggested in addition to established cardiac therapy. The symphony of cardiovascular health contains not just pharmacological notes, but also the harmonic chords of lifestyle changes coordinated with vagus nerve stimulation.

Collaborations between conventional and alternative medicine

- **Holistic health clinics and integrated care:**

The incorporation of vagus nerve methods is particularly apparent in holistic health clinics and integrative care settings. Traditional and alternative medicine practitioners work together to build a dynamic ensemble. Physicians, acupuncturists, naturopaths, and psychologists collaborate to offer holistic treatment that addresses the many facets of health.

- **Vagus Nerve Stimulation Devices in Mainstream Care**

Medical technological advancements, such as vagus nerve stimulation devices, help to facilitate integration. Epilepsy and depression are treated using FDA-approved devices that stimulate the vagus nerve. The convergence of technology and traditional healing practices connects alternative treatments with evidence-based medicine.

Optimal Results from Comprehensive Approaches

- **Individualised treatment plans:**
The integration of vagus nerve procedures takes place in the context of specific treatment regimens. Recognizing that each person's health journey is unique, healthcare practitioners work together to customise therapies. These programs include vagus nerve procedures, which give people with skills for self-care and empowerment.

- **Combining pharmaceuticals and holistic practices:**

In circumstances when pharmacological treatments are required, the integration goes beyond mixing drugs with holistic therapies. Individuals on antidepressants, for example, may be advised to use mindfulness activities to improve the therapeutic benefits. This collaborative strategy seeks to achieve best outcomes while reducing adverse effects.

- **Preventive Health and Lifestyle Medicine.**

The integration goes beyond treating current illnesses to include preventative health and lifestyle medicine. Nutrition, exercise, and stress-reduction approaches based on vagus nerve stimulation are used to improve holistic well-being. This proactive approach targets the underlying causes of health issues, developing resilience and avoiding the genesis of certain illnesses.

Opportunities and Challenges in Integration

- **Paradigm shifts provide the following challenges**:

The incorporation of vagus nerve procedures into contemporary medicine is not without difficulties. Paradigm transformations, both within the medical establishment and among patients, take time and effort. Scepticism may occur, forcing attempts to bridge the divide between conventional and alternative viewpoints. Overcoming these obstacles requires open communication about the data supporting vagus nerve therapies and their place within a larger healthcare framework.

- **Opportunities for holistic healing:**

Opportunities for holistic healing develop in the face of obstacles. Integrating vagus nerve treatments facilitates a more patient-centred, holistic approach to healthcare. It supports a move away from symptom-focused therapies and toward addressing the root causes of health imbalances. Individuals may actively engage in their recovery journeys because of integration, which fosters a feeling of agency and connectedness to their well-being.

Chapter 13

Unlocking the physical resilience within: the vagus nerve's role beyond mental health

In the complicated tapestry of well-being, the vagus nerve emerges as a major thread—a conductor directing both the symphony of emotions and the nuanced ballet of physiological reactions. Beyond its well-known function in mental health, the vagus nerve has a significant impact on physical resilience, notably in the complex dance of cardiovascular health. This investigation dives into the vagus nerve symphony, revealing its effects on the cardiovascular system and the entire picture of physical well-being.

The Cardiovascular Ballet: A Harmony Conducted By the Vagus Nerve

▪ Understanding Cardiovascular Connection:

The circulatory system, with its complicated network of veins and the repetitive beating of the heart, creates a stage for the vagus nerve to perform a dance of balance. The vagus nerve, an important component of the autonomic nervous system, regulates heart function in complex ways. Its branches weave through the heart's fabric, regulating the rate, rhythm, and general harmony of circulatory activity.

▪ Heart rate variability as a measure of resilience:

Heart rate variability (HRV) is a major measure of the vagus nerve's effect on cardiovascular health. HRV monitors fluctuations in the time interval between subsequent heartbeats, indicating the cardiovascular system's flexibility and resilience. Higher HRV is related with greater cardiovascular health, reflecting the system's ability to adapt to shifting demands.

Cardiovascular Harmony via Vagus Nerve Activation

- **Impact on heart rate and blood pressure:**
The symphony of vagus nerve activity is reflected in the regulation of heart rate and blood pressure. As the vagus nerve moves

with the heart, it reduces the pace, allowing for a more deliberate and regulated beat. At the same time, it interacts delicately with blood vessels, modulating their tone and controlling blood pressure. This synchronisation creates a circulatory environment that supports resilience and good performance.

- **Anti-inflammatory Serenade**

The cardiovascular ballet goes beyond the beating of the heart and the flow of blood. When the vagus nerve is active, it performs an anti-inflammatory serenade. It interacts with the immune system, reducing the inflammatory response that may lead to the development and progression of cardiovascular disease. This anti-inflammatory regulation becomes an important note in the orchestration of cardiovascular resilience.

Beyond the Heartbeat: Physical Resilience Increased

- **The Digestive Symphony:**

The vagus nerve's effect extends beyond the circulatory stage, including the digestive system in a symphony of synchronised activity. Activation of the vagus nerve improves digestion processes by increasing enzyme production and enhancing nutrition absorption. This intestinal harmony benefits not just gut health but also general physical resilience by ensuring the body obtains the nutrients it needs for energy and repairs.

- **Respiratory Rhythm:**

The respiratory system contributes to the vagus nerve's symphony of physical resilience. Deep, diaphragmatic breathing, which is a sign of vagus nerve activity, promotes respiratory rhythms that go beyond basic oxygen exchange. It sets off a series of physiological reactions, including respiratory muscle relaxation and the release of calming neurotransmitters. This respiratory dance improves general physical health by encouraging relaxation and lowering the physiological imprint of stress.

The Stress-Resilience Connection: A Harmony of Hormones

- **Balancing the stress hormones:**

The vagus nerve's effect on physical resilience is linked to its control of stress chemicals. When faced with stimuli, the sympathetic nervous system engages the "fight or flight" response, producing stress chemicals such as cortisol and adrenaline. The vagus nerve, functioning as a balancer, activates the parasympathetic nervous system, signifying the restoration of calm and equilibrium. This hormonal balance promotes resilience by limiting prolonged activation of stress reactions, which may lead to a variety of physical health problems.

Physical Resilience Outside of the Individual: The Immune Ensemble

- **Immune System Symphony**

The vagus nerve exerts its impact on the immune system, orchestrating immunological responses. The vagus nerve interacts with immune cells, regulating their activity and supporting a healthy immunological response. This coordination keeps the immune system alert against infections while preventing excessive inflammation, which contributes to general physical resilience.

▪ Increasing Physical Resilience Through Vagus Nerve Activation:

▪ Holistic Well-Being as the Crescendo

Cultivating physical resilience via vagus nerve activation goes beyond individual treatments. It culminates in a harmonious synthesis of lifestyle habits, thoughtful decisions, and deliberate use of vagus nerve treatments. This well-being symphony includes aspects such as regular physical exercise, a nutritious diet, enough sleep, and stress-management techniques that are linked to vagus nerve activation.

▪ Adopting a Vagus Nerve-Friendly Lifestyle

Physical resilience encourages people to have a vagus nerve-friendly lifestyle. This includes smoothly incorporating vagus nerve therapies into regular routines, such as morning mindfulness sessions and attentive breathing pauses throughout the day. Engaging in activities that promote pleasure, appreciation, and connection increases the vibrancy of the vagus nerve's symphony, which contributes to physical strength.

Challenges and Opportunities for Increasing Physical Resilience:

- **The challenges of modern lifestyles:**
Modern lifestyle demands provide obstacles in the current orchestration of well-being. Sedentary behaviours, persistent stresses, and poor nutritional choices may all disrupt the symphony of physical resilience. Addressing these difficulties requires a

deliberate effort to realign daily routines with activities that promote vagus nerve activation and general physical well-being.

- **Opportunities For Empowerment:**

Challenges include chances for empowerment. Increasing physical resilience via vagus nerve stimulation encourages people to become active participants in their health journey. Educating people about the importance of the vagus nerve and offering practical strategies for activating it allows them to create resilience in the face of life's challenges.

Conclusion: Embracing the melody within: A harmonious conclusion on the transformative power of the vagus nerve

As we pull the curtains on our investigation into the vagus nerve's transformational ability, the tune's resonance lingers—a melody that crosses mental and physical borders, creating a tapestry of well-being. In this last part, we'll summarise the vagus nerve's symphony of change and invite readers to discover and embrace the activities that unleash its tremendous potential.

- **Recapitulating the transformative journey:**

The vagus nerve, sometimes known as the "wandering nerve," travels on a transforming trip that reaches the very centre of our existence. From its function in mental health, where it orchestrates the symphony of emotions and stress reactions, to its complicated tango with the cardiovascular system, which influences heart rate, blood pressure, and general resilience, the vagus nerve emerges as a conductor of total well-being.

In terms of physical resilience, the vagus nerve exerts its impact via synchronising heartbeats, breathing patterns, and immunological responses. Its influence extends beyond the person, resonating with the interwoven symphony of the mind, emotion, and body. As a brain maestro, the vagus nerve promotes balance, resilience, and vitality—a song that resonates across the complexities of our physiological and emotional landscapes.

■ Encouragement to explore and embrace:

As we approach the conclusion of this transforming trip, we offer an invitation to each reader to study and embrace the techniques that activate the vagus nerve's hidden potential. Consider it an invitation to join the symphony, to take an active role in the dance of well-being, and to tap into your own innate ability for healing and resilience.

▪ Delving into Vagus Nerve Practices:
Beginning this investigation entails researching vagus nerve activities that are compatible with individual tastes and lifestyles. The vagus nerve therapies are various, ranging from basic but effective

deep breathing exercises to the calming melodies of meditation and awareness. It invites exploration, allowing people to find activities that work with their specific rhythms.

- **Incorporating into Daily Life:**

The vagus nerve transforming capacity is most effective when it is seamlessly incorporated into everyday activities that promote a vagus nerve-friendly lifestyle. Whether it's a moment of awareness during the morning sunrise, a mindful breathing break in the middle of a hectic day, or the regular cadence of a contemplative practice before sleep, these moments become notes in a continuing symphony of well-being.

- **Final Notes of Empowerment:**

Allow the tones of empowerment to echo in the final movement. The vagus nerve's transformational potential goes beyond the pages of this book and into each reader's own experiences. It is an invitation to take control of one's own health, to accept the conductor's baton, and to become the orchestrator of one's own symphony.

As the vagus nerve symphony continues, allow it to be a source of inspiration, resilience, and healing. May the transformational voyage, led by the wandering nerve's music, serve as a tribute to each person's intrinsic ability to reset, activate, and triumph over the hardships of contemporary life.

In the grand climax of this journey, the curtain falls with a thunderous echo, carrying the harmonising vibrations of the vagus nerve's transforming ability. As you embrace the song inside, may your journey with the vagus nerve be a never-ending symphony—a melody that develops with each breath, echoes with each heartbeat, and leads to a life in tune with the inherent potential for completeness and well-being.

Thank you for reading one of my books! Your Feedback Is Valuable! Have you savoured the voyage utilising the vagus nerve's transformative potential? Please provide your feedback by leaving a review. We are guided by your insights as we create topics that are more beneficial to you. We highly regard your experience; by sharing it with us, you will contribute to our ongoing development.